Keto C

Recipes Cookbook

50 Quick and Easy Ketogenic

Waffles to Lose Weight in an

Healthy Way

By Rita Adams

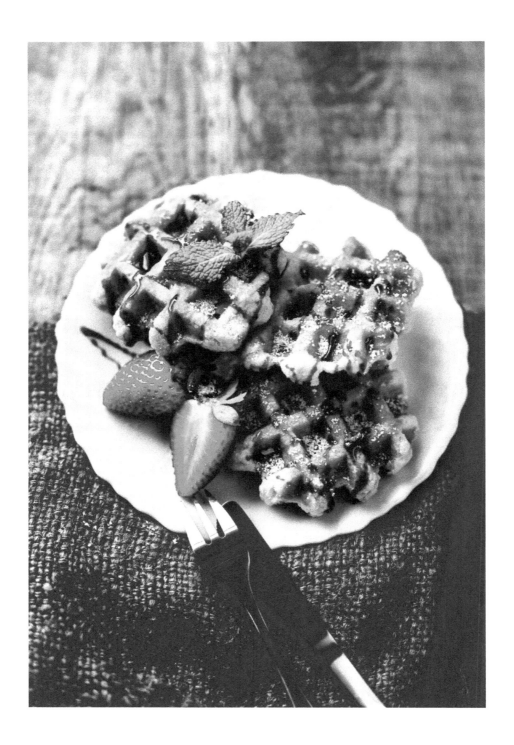

Table of Contents

Chapter 3: Savory Recipes 48

Chapter 4: Vegan and Vegetarian Recipes 76

Additionally, the information in the following pages is intended only for informational purposes and should thus be thought of as universal. As befitting its nature, it is presented without assurance regarding its prolonged validity or interim quality. Trademarks that are mentioned are done without written consent and can in no way be considered an endorsement from the trademark holder.

Introduction

Chaffle

We present to you the "Chaffle" or "cheddar waffle", an extremely delicious waffle you can easily prepare at home, but made with egg and butter as base ingredients instead of grain, they are perfect to stay in ketosis as shredded cheese have no flour.

The high flour content in regular waffles adds a lot of carbohydrates that makes your body stop using fat as an energy resource, and consequently start accumulating it, due to spikes in your insulin levels caused by the carb intake.

This healthy food, that follow the ketogenic diet recommendations, will also keep you feeling full for a long time as they are high-fat and high-protein, preventing overeating, they are a great alternative for bread, perfect in their simplicity.

You can enjoy this mouth-watering dish in every meal of your day, there are countless combinations of low-carb ketogenic ingredients aviable, so it's easy to find a chaffle one to love!

Depending on how you serve them, they can be delicious sweet desserts, nutrient breakfast food or a quick snack, try them in sandiwhich, pizza and French toast variations!

The best option to make them is the Chaffle Maker, but you can prepare yourself one with a regular Waffle maker or even a nonstick saucepan.

Some people does not like the taste that comes from the egg as a base ingredients, here some tips on how to avoid too much eggy taste:
-Increase the sugar quantity
-Add milk powder
-Add Lime, lemon, or orange juice. Use a teaspoon of juice per 3 eggs
-Add some rind. Use quarter teaspoon per 3 eggs.
-Let chaffle cool completely
-Use egg whites instead of whole eggs

Note

> You can freeze them up for 3 to 5 days and then reheat them in a toaster oven, skillet, or conventional oven.

> You can also microwave for 30 to 60 seconds, but allow them to thaw before reheating.

> You can make two chaffles from a large egg and half a cup of shredded cheese.

> Not every type pf cheese is totally carb free.
> If using the cream cheese melt or soft it, before stirring it into the batter.

- ➤ If using coconut flour, let the batter sit for 2-3 minutes to thicken up.

- ➤ It's better to use finely shredded cheese for the batter.

- ➤ To make your chaffle crispier sprinkle some extra cheese in the waffle iron before adding the batter.

- ➤ Do not open the waffle iron too early to check it. It should continue cooking until the chaffle is done and crisp. Let it cook for slightly longer for best results. It's best to cook most of the chaffle recipes for a minimum of 4 minutes, in general you will know the chaffle is ready when steam is no longer coming out of the sides.

- ➤ Mozzarella is always the best option because thanks to its mildness and it is not as greasy as many other cheese varieties.

- ➤ If you are using a nonstick saucepan to make your chaffles, grease and hot the pan before pouring the batter, then let it cook until golden brown and use a spatula to gently flip it.

Chaffle Maker

- ➤ There are many brands available, each with different cooking times and non-stick versions.

- Make sure that the surface is not too hot before you clean the waffle or chaffle maker.

- Use a damp cloth or paper towel for wiping away the crumbs.

- Soak up the excess oil drips on your grid plates.

- Wipe the exterior with the damp cloth or paper towel.

- Pour a few drops of cooking oil on the batter to remove the stubborn batter drips. Allow it to sit for a few minutes. Then wipe it away.

- Ensure that the waffle maker is completely dry before storing it.

- Always read the instruction manual before you use it for the first time.

- Just a light cooking oil coating is enough for nonstick waffle makers.

- Grease the grid with a little amount of oil if you see the waffles sticking.
- Never use metal or sharp tools to scrape off the batter or to remove the cooked waffles. You may end up scratching the surface and damaging it.

- Do not submerge your electric waffle maker in water.

➢ Clean the chaffle maker as soon as it is cool enough;

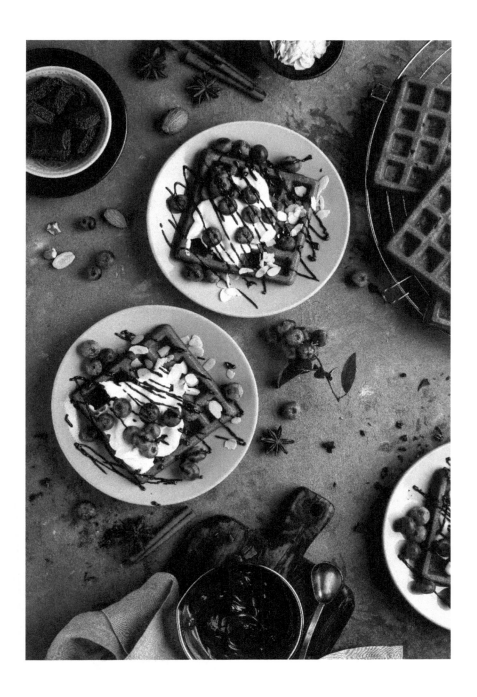

Chapter 1: Basic Chaffle Recipes

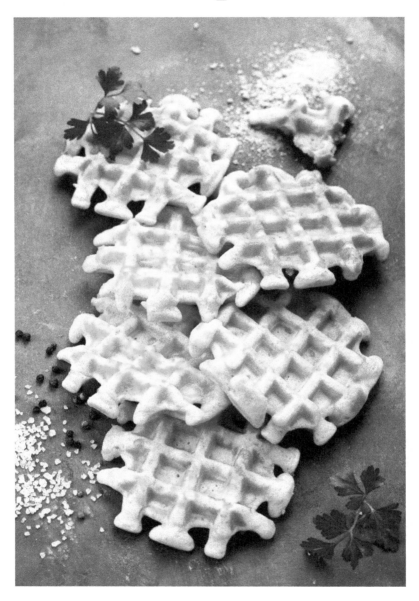

Basic Recipe for Cheese Chaffles

Preparation: 6 minutes | Cooking: 15 minutes | Servings: 2

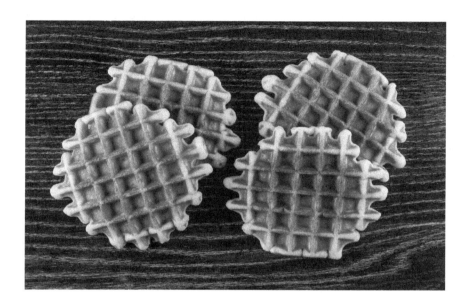

Ingredients

- 1 medium or large egg
- 50 g of grated Mozzarella (fresh, self-grated is less suitable) cheese butter
- Salt
- Pepper

Directions

1. While the chaffle iron is heating, whisk the egg and then fold in the fresh mozzarella.
2. Season with pepper and salt and add a little butter to the iron. As soon as it is melted and well distributed, add the dough and bake the cheese chaffles until they are golden

brown and crispy. Salty chaffles of this type taste both warm and cold.

Nutrition: Calories 126, Fat 4.3, Fiber 2.1, Carbs 9.1, Protein 5.2

Almonds and Flaxseeds Chaffles

Preparation: 10 minutes | Cooking: 5 minutes | Servings: 2

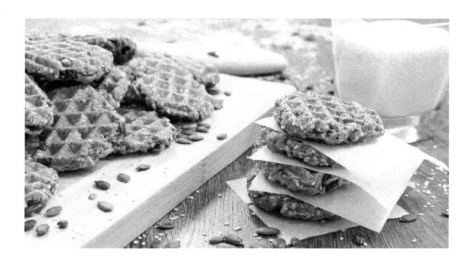

Ingredients

- 1/4 cup coconut flour
- 1 tsp. stevia
- 1 tbsp. ground flaxseed
- 1/4 tsp. baking powder
- 1/2 cup almond milk
- 1/4 tsp. vanilla extract
- 1/ cup low carb vegan cheese

Directions

1. Mix together flaxseed in warm water and set aside.
2. Add in the remaining ingredients.
3. Switch on waffle iron and grease with cooking spray.
4. Pour the batter in the waffle machine and close the lid.

5. Cooking the chaffles for about 3-4 minutes.
6. Once cooked, remove from the waffle machine.
7. Serve with berries and enjoy!

Nutrition: Calories per | Servings: 371; Carbohydrates: 6.4g; Protein: 40.7g; Fat: 24.1g; Sugar: 0g; Sodium: 720mg; Fiber: 3.9g

Vegan Chaffles With Flaxseed

Preparation: 10 minutes | Cooking: 5 minutes | Servings: 2

Ingredients

- 1 tbsp. flaxseed meal
- 2 tbsps. warm water
- ¼ cup low carb vegan cheese
- ¼ cup chopped minutest
- pinch of salt
- 2 oz. blueberries chunks

Directions

1. Preheat waffle maker to medium-high heat and grease with cooking spray.
2. Mix together flaxseed meal and warm water and set aside to be thickened.
3. After 5 minutes' mix together all ingredients in flax egg.
4. Pour vegan waffle batter into the center of the waffle iron.
5. Close the waffle maker and let cooking for 3-minutes
6. Once cooked, remove the vegan chaffle from the waffle maker and serve.

Nutrition: 295 Calories, 21g Protein, 7.2g Carbohydrates, 21.1g Fat, 1.9g Fiber, 69mg Cholesterol, 569mg Sodium, 118mg Potassium

Rosemary Chaffle

Preparation: 5 minutes | Cooking: 8 minutes | Servings: 2 chaffles

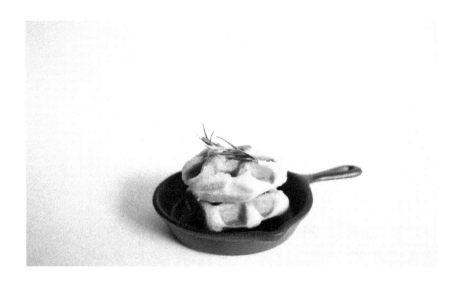

Ingredients

- 1 egg, beaten
- ½ cup shredded cheddar cheese
- ½ tbsp fresh rosemary, finely chopped

Directions

1. Heat up the waffle maker.
2. Add egg, shredded cheddar cheese, and rosemary to a small mixing bowl and combine well.
3. Pour half of the batter into the waffle maker and cook for 4 minutes until brown. Repeat with the rest of the batter to make another chaffle.
4. Serve with your favorite keto dressing and enjoy!

Cinnamon Keto Chaffles

Preparation: 5 minutes | Cooking: 10 minutes | Servings: 3

Ingredients

- 1/2 cup Mozzarella cheese
- 1 tablespoon almond flour
- 1/4 tsp. baking powder
- 1 egg
- 1 tsp. cinnamon
- 1 tsp. Granulated Swerve

Cinnamon roll swirl:

- 1 tbsp. butter
- 1 tsp. cinnamon
- 2 tsp. confectioner's swerve

Keto Cinnamon Roll Glaze:

- 1 tablespoon butter
- 1 tablespoon cream cheese
- 1/4 tsp. vanilla extract
- 2 tsp. swerve confectioners

Directions

1. Plug in your Mini Dash Waffle maker and let it heat up.
2. In a small bowl mix the Mozzarella cheese, almond flour, baking powder, egg, 1 teaspoon cinnamon, and 1 teaspoon swerve granulated and set aside.

3. In another small bowl, add a tablespoon of butter, 1 teaspoon cinnamon, and 2 teaspoons of swerve confectioners' sweetener.
4. Microwave for 15 seconds and mix well.
5. Spray the waffle maker with nonstick spray and add 1/3 of the batter to your waffle maker. Swirl in 1/3 of the cinnamon, swerve, and butter mixture onto the top of it. Close the waffle maker and let cooking for 3-4 minutes.
6. When the first cinnamon roll chaffle is done, make the second and then make the third.
7. While the third chaffle is cooking place 1 tablespoon butter and 1 tablespoon of cream cheese in a small bowl. Heat in the microwave for 10-15 seconds. Start at 10, and if the cream cheese is not soft enough to mix with the butter heat for an additional 5 seconds.
8. Add the vanilla extract, and the swerve confectioner's sweetener to the butter and cream cheese and mix well using a whisk.
9. Drizzle keto cream cheese glaze on top of chaffle.

Nutrition: Calories: 370g, Fat: 26g, Carbs: 5g, Protein: 25g.

Keto Chaffle Stuffing Recipe

Preparation: 5 minutes | Cooking: 12 minutes | Servings: 4

Ingredients

Basic Chaffle:

- 1/2 cup cheese mozzarella, cheddar or a combo of both
- 2 eggs
- 1/4 tsp. garlic powder
- 1/2 tsp. onion powder
- 1/2 tsp. dried poultry seasoning
- 1/4 tsp. salt
- 1/4 tsp. pepper

Stuffing:

- 1 small onion diced
- 2 celery stalks
- 4 oz. mushrooms diced
- 4 tbs butter for sauteing
- 3 eggs

Directions

1. First, make your chaffles.
2. Preheat the mini waffle iron.
3. Preheat the oven to 350F
4. In a medium-size bowl, combine the chaffle ingredients.
5. Pour a 1/4 of the mixture into a mini waffle maker and cooking each chaffle for about 4 minutes each.
6. Once they are all cooked, set them aside.

7. In a small frying pan, sauté the onion, celery, and mushrooms until they are soft.
8. In a separate bowl, tear up the chaffles into small pieces, add the sauteed veggies, and 3 eggs. Mix until the ingredients are fully combined.
9. Add the stuffing mixture to a small casserole dish (about a 4 x 4) and bake it at 350 degrees for about 30 to 40 minutes.

Nutrition: Calories: 298, Fat: 17g, Carbs: 7,2, Protein: 23g.

Chaffle Churros

Preparation: 10 min. | Cooking: 5 min. | Servings: 2

Ingredients

- 1 egg
- 1 Tbsp. almond flour
- ½ tsp. vanilla extract
- 1 tsp. cinnamon, divided
- ¼ tsp. baking powder
- ½ cup shredded mozzarella
- 1 Tbsp. swerve confectioners' sugar substitute
- 1 Tbsp. swerve brown sugar substitute
- 1 Tbsp. butter, melted

Directions

1. Turn on waffle maker to heat and oil it with cooking spray.
2. Mix egg, flour, vanilla extract, ½ tsp. cinnamon, baking powder, mozzarella, and sugar substitute in a bowl.
3. Place half of the mixture into waffle maker and cooking for 3-5 minutes, or until desired doneness. Remove and place the second half of the batter into the maker.
4. Cut chaffles into strips.
5. Place strips in a bowl and cover with melted butter.
6. Mix brown sugar substitute and the remaining cinnamon in a bowl. Pour sugar mixture over the strips and toss to coat them well.

Nutrition: Calories: 372, Fat: 16g, Carbs: 3g, Protein: 40g.

Cocoa Chaffles

Preparation: 5 min. | Cooking: 5 min. | Servings: 2

Ingredients

- 1 egg
- 1½ Tbsp. unsweetened cocoa
- 2 Tbsp. lakanto monk fruit, or choice of sweetener
- 1 Tbsp. heavy cream
- 1 tsp. coconut flour
- ½ tsp. baking powder
- ½ tsp. vanilla

For the Cheese Cream:

- 1 Tbsp. lakanto powdered sweetener
- 2 Tbsp. softened cream cheese
- ¼ tsp. vanilla

Directions

1. Turn on waffle maker to heat and oil it with cooking spray. Combine all chaffle ingredients in a small bowl.
2. Pour one half of the chaffle mixture into waffle maker. Cooking for 3-5 minutes.
3. Remove and repeat with the second half if the mixture. Let chaffles sit for 2-3 to crisp up.
4. Combine all cream ingredients and spread on chaffle when they have cooled to room temperature.

Nutrition: Calories: 343g. Fat: 27g, Carbs: 4g, Protein: 21g

Fresh Dill Chaffle

Preparation: 5 minutes | Cooking: 8 minutes | Servings: 2 chaffles

Ingredients

- 1 egg, beaten
- ½ cup shredded cheddar cheese
- ½ tbsp fresh dill, finely chopped

Directions

1. Heat up the waffle maker.
2. Add egg, shredded cheddar cheese, and dill to a small mixing bowl and combine well.
3. Pour half of the batter into the waffle maker and cook for 4 minutes until brown. Repeat with the rest of the batter to make another chaffle.
4. Serve with your favorite keto dressing and enjoy!

Fresh Coriander Chaffle

Preparation: 5 minutes | Cooking: 8 minutes | Servings: 2 chaffles

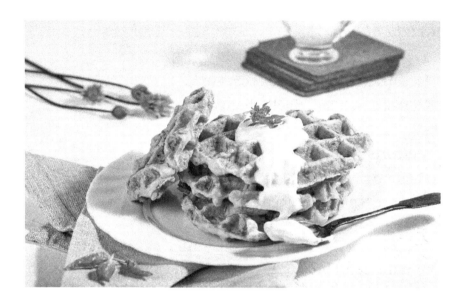

Ingredients

- 1 egg, beaten
- ½ cup shredded mozzarella cheese
- 1 tsp coconut flour
- ¼ tsp baking powder
- ½ tsp fresh coriander, minced

Directions

1. Heat up the waffle maker.
2. Add all the ingredients to a small mixing bowl and combine well.

3. Pour half of the batter into the waffle maker and cook for 4 minutes until golden brown. Repeat with the rest of the batter to make another chaffle.
4. Let cool for 3 minutes to let chaffles get crispy.
5. Serve and enjoy!

Chapter 2: Breakfast and Brunch Recipes

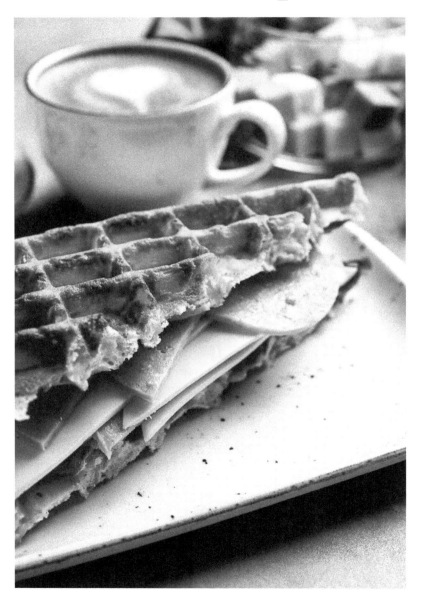

Fluffy Sandwich Breakfast Chaffle

Preparation: 5 min | Cooking: 3 min | Servings: 2

Ingredients
- 1/2 tsp Psyllium husk powder (optional)
- tbsp almond flour
- 1/4 tsp Baking powder (optional)
- 1 large Egg
- 1/2 cup Mozzarella cheese, shredded
- 1 tbsp vanilla or
- Dash of cinnamon

Directions:
1. Switch on the waffle maker according to manufacturer's Directions
2. Crack egg and combine with cheddar cheese in a small bowl
3. Add remaining ingredients and combine thoroughly.
4. Place half batter on waffle maker and spread evenly.
5. Cook for 4 minutes or until as desired
6. Gently remove from waffle maker and set aside for 2 minutes so it cools down and become crispy
7. Repeat for remaining batter
8. Serve with keto ice cream topping

Scrambled Eggs and A Spring Onion Chaffle

Preparation: 10 minutes | Cooking: 7–9 Minutes | Servings: 4

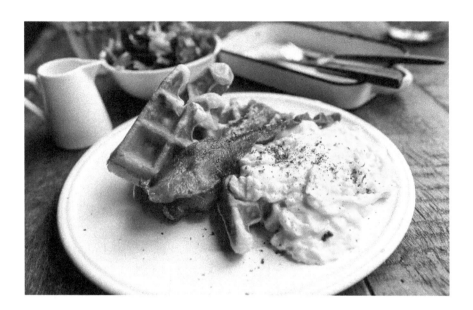

Ingredients

Batter:

- 4 eggs
- 2 cups grated Mozzarella cheese
- 2 spring onions, finely chopped
- Salt and pepper to taste
- ½ teaspoon dried garlic powder
- 2 tablespoons almond flour
- 2 tablespoons coconut flour

Other:

- 2 tablespoons butter for brushing the waffle maker
- 6-8 eggs
- Salt and pepper
- 1 teaspoon Italian spice mix
- 1 tablespoon olive oil
- 1 tablespoon freshly chopped parsley

Directions

1. Preheat the waffle maker.
2. Crack the eggs into a bowl and add the grated cheese.
3. Mix until just combined, then add the chopped spring onions and season with salt and pepper and dried garlic powder.
4. Stir in the almond flour and mix until everything is combined.
5. Brush the heated waffle maker with butter and add a few tablespoons of the batter.
6. Close the lid and cooking for about 7–8 minutes depending on your waffle maker.
7. While the chaffles are cooking, prepare the scrambled eggs by whisking the eggs in a bowl until frothy, about 2 minutes. Season with salt and black pepper to taste and add the Italian spice mix. Whisk to blend in the spices.
8. Warm the oil in a non-stick pan over medium heat.
9. Pour the eggs in the pan and cooking until eggs are set to your liking.
10. Serve each chaffle and top with some scrambled eggs. Top with freshly chopped parsley.

Nutrition: Calories: 165; Total Fat: 15g; Carbs: 4g; Net Carbs: 2g; Fiber: 2g; Protein: 6g

Egg and A Cheddar Cheese Chaffle

Preparation: 10 minutes | Cooking: 7–9 Minutes | Servings: 4

Ingredients

Batter:

- 4 eggs
- 2 cups shredded white cheddar cheese
- Salt and pepper to taste

Other:

- 2 tablespoons butter for brushing the waffle maker
- 4 large eggs
- 2 tablespoons olive oil

Directions

1. Preheat the waffle maker.
2. Crack the eggs into a bowl and whisk them with a fork.
3. Stir in the grated cheddar cheese and season with salt and pepper.
4. Brush the heated waffle maker with butter and add a few tablespoons of the batter.
5. Close the lid and cooking for about 7–8 minutes depending on your waffle maker.
6. While chaffles are cooking, cooking the eggs.
7. Warm the oil in a large non-stick pan that has a lid over medium-low heat for 2-3 minutes
8. Crack an egg in a small ramekin and gently add it to the pan. Repeat the same way for the other 3 eggs.

9. Cover and let cooking for 2 to 2 ½ minutes for set eggs but with runny yolks.
10. Remove from heat.
11. To serve, place a chaffle on each plate and top with an egg. Season with salt and black pepper to taste.

Nutrition: Calories: 74; Total Fat: 7g; Carbs: 1g; Net Carbs: 0g; Fiber: 0g; Protein: 3g

Celery and Cottage Cheese Chaffle

Preparation: 10 minutes | Cooking: 15 minutes | Servings: 4

Ingredients

- 4 eggs
- 2 cups grated cheddar cheese
- 1 cup fresh celery, chopped
- Salt and pepper to taste
- 2 tablespoons chopped almonds
- 2 teaspoons baking powder
- 2 tablespoons cooking spray to brush the waffle maker ¼ cup cottage cheese for serving

Directions

1. Preheat the waffle maker.
2. Add the eggs, grated Mozzarella cheese, chopped celery, salt and pepper, chopped almonds and baking powder to a bowl.
3. Mix with a fork.
4. Brush the heated waffle maker with cooking spray and add a few tablespoons of the batter.
5. Close the lid and cooking for about 7 minutes depending on your waffle maker.
6. Serve each chaffle with cottage cheese on top.

Nutrition: Calories 292, Fat 12, Fiber 3, Carbs 7, Protein 16

Mushroom and Almond Chaffle

Preparation: 10 minutes | Cooking: 15 minutes | Servings: 4

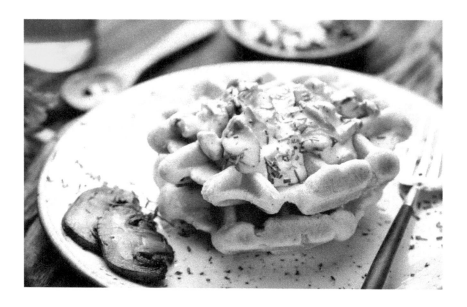

Ingredients

- 4 eggs
- 2 cups grated Mozzarella cheese
- 1 cup finely chopped zucchini
- 3 tablespoons chopped almonds
- 2 teaspoons baking powder
- Salt and pepper to taste
- 1 teaspoon dried basil
- 1 teaspoon chili flakes
- 2 tablespoons cooking spray to brush the waffle maker

Directions

1. Preheat the waffle maker.

2. Add the eggs, grated mozzarella, mushrooms, almonds, baking powder, salt and pepper, dried basil and chili flakes to a bowl.
3. Mix with a fork.
4. Brush the heated waffle maker with cooking spray and add a few tablespoons of the batter.
5. Close the lid and cooking for about 7 minutes depending on your waffle maker.
6. Serve and enjoy.

Nutrition: Calories 254, Fat 12, Fiber 3, Carbs 6, Protein 16

Spinach and Artichoke Chaffle

Preparation: 10 minutes | Cooking: 15 minutes | Servings: 4

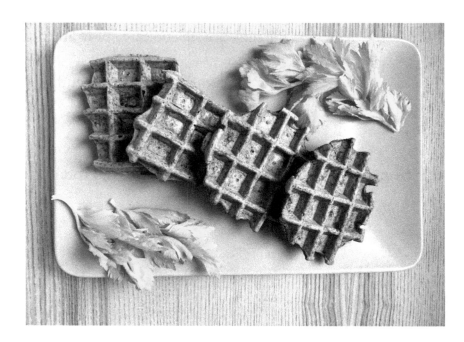

Ingredients

- 4 eggs
- 2 cups grated provolone cheese
- 1 cup cooked and diced spinach
- ½ cup diced artichoke hearts
- Salt and pepper to taste
- 2 tablespoons coconut flour
- 2 teaspoons baking powder
- 2 tablespoons cooking spray to brush the waffle maker
- ¼ cup of cream cheese for serving

Directions

1. Preheat the waffle maker.
2. Add the eggs, grated provolone cheese, diced spinach, artichoke hearts, salt and pepper, coconut flour and baking powder to a bowl.
3. Mix with a fork.
4. Brush the heated waffle maker with cooking spray and add a few tablespoons of the batter.
5. Close the lid and cooking for about 7 minutes depending on your waffle maker.
6. Serve each chaffle with cream cheese.

Nutrition: Calories 250, Fat 5, Fiber 7, Carbs 15, Protein 20

Chaffles Breakfast Bowl

Preparation: 15 min | Cooking: 5 min | Servings: 2

Ingredients:

- 1 egg
- 1/2 cup cheddar cheese shredded
- pinch of Italian seasoning
- 1 tbsp. pizza sauce
- 1/2 avocado sliced
- 2 eggs boiled
- 1 tomato, halves
- 4 oz. fresh spinach leaves

Directions

1. Preheat your waffle maker and grease with cooking spray.
2. Crack an egg in a small bowl and beat with Italian seasoning and pizza sauce.
3. Add shredded cheese to the egg and spices mixture.
4. Pour 1 tbsp. shredded cheese in a waffle maker and cooking for 30 sec.
5. Pour Chaffles batter in the waffle maker and close the lid.
6. Cooking chaffles for about 4 minutes until crispy and brown.
7. Carefully remove chaffles from the maker.
8. Serve on the bed of spinach with boil egg, avocado slice, and tomatoes.
9. Enjoy!

Nutrition: Calories: 549; Total Fat: 49g; Carbs: 16g; Net Carbs: 11g:
Fiber: 5g; Protein: 16g

Mini Breakfast Chaffles

Preparation: 5 Min | Cooking: 15 Min | Servings: 3

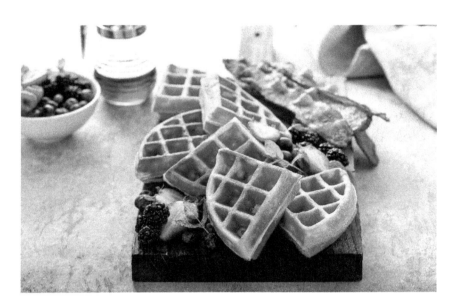

Ingredients

- 6 tsp coconut flour
- 1 tsp stevia
- 1/4 tsp baking powder
- 2 eggs
- 3 oz. cream cheese
- 1/2. tsp vanilla extract

Topping:

- 1 egg
- 6 slice bacon
- 2 oz. Raspberries for topping
- 2 oz. Blueberries for topping

- 2 oz. Strawberries for topping

Directions

1. Heat up your square waffle maker and grease with cooking spray.
2. Mix together coconut flour, stevia, egg, baking powder, cheese and vanilla in mixing bowl.
3. Pour ½ of chaffles mixture in a waffle maker.
4. Close the lid and cook the chaffles for about 3-5 minutes.
5. Meanwhile, fry bacon slices in pan on medium heat for about 2-3 minutes until cooked and transfer themto plate.
6. In the same pan, fry eggs one by one in the leftover grease of bacon.
7. Once chaffles are cooked, carefully transferthem toplate.
8. Serve with fried eggs and bacon slice and berries on top.
9. Enjoy!

Zucchini & Basil Chaffles

Cooking: 10 Minutes | Servings: 2

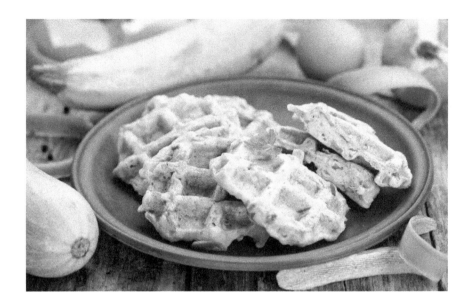

Ingredients

- 1 organic egg, beaten
- 1/4 cup Mozzarella cheese, shredded
- 2 tablespoons Parmesan cheese, grated
- 1/2 of small zucchini, grated and squeezed
- 1/4 teaspoon dried basil, crushed
- Freshly ground black pepper, as required

Directions

1. Preheat a mini waffle iron and then grease it.
2. In a medium bowl, place all ingredients and mix until well combined.

3. Place half of the mixture into preheated waffle iron and cook for about 4-5 minutes or until golden brown.
4. Repeat with the remaining mixture.
5. Serve warm.

Nutrition: Net Carb: 1g, Fat: 4.1g, Saturated Fat: 1.7g, Carbohydrates:1.3g , Dietary Fiber: 0.3g, Sugar: 0.7g, Protein: 6.1g

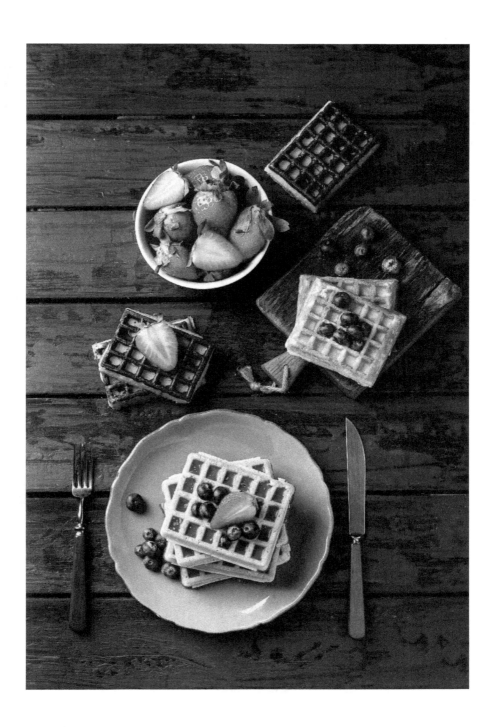

Chapter 3: Savory Recipes

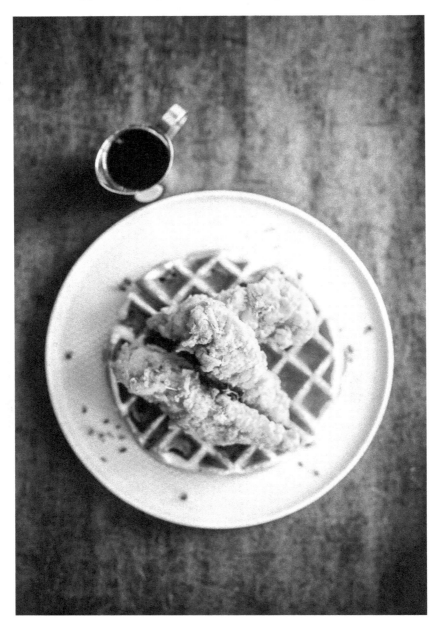

Israelian Chaffle

Preparation: 10 minutes | Cooking: 20 minutes | Servings: 4 chaffles

Ingridients

For chaffles:

- 2 large eggs, beaten
- 1 cup cheddar cheese, shredded
- 2 scallions, minced
- A pinch of salt and pepper

For topping:

- 2 chicken breasts, cooked and shredded
- ¼ cup keto buffalo sauce
- 3 tbsp keto hummus
- 2 celery stalks, minced
- ¼ cup cheddar cheese, shredded

Directions:

1. Heat up the waffle maker and preheat oven at 400°.
2. In a mixing bowl add hummus, chicken, sauce and celery stalks. Combine well and set aside.
3. Add all the chaffles ingredients in a separate mixing bowl and stir until well combined.
4. Pour ¼ of the batter into the waffle maker and cook for 4 minutes until golden brown. Repeat with the rest of the batter to prepare the other chaffles.

5. Arrange the chaffles in the baking sheet lined with parchment paper.
6. Top each chaffle with the chicken mixture and sprinkle with cheddar cheese.
7. Bake for approx. 5 minutes or until the cheese bubbles.
8. Serve and enjoy!

Spicy Jalapeno & Bacon Chaffles

Preparation: 5 Minutes | Cooking: 5 Minutes | Servings: 2

Ingredients

- 1 oz. cream cheese
- 1 large egg
- 1/2 cup cheddar cheese
- 2 tbsps. bacon bits
- 1/2 tbsp. jalapenos
- 1/4 tsp baking powder

Directions

1. Switch on your waffle maker.
2. Grease your waffle maker with cooking spray and let it heat up.
3. Mix together egg and vanilla extract in a bowl first.
4. Add baking powder, jalapenos and bacon bites.
5. Add in cheese last and mix together.
6. Pour the chaffles batter intothe maker and cook the chaffles for about 2-3 minutes.
7. Once chaffles are cooked, remove from the maker.
8. Serve hot and enjoy!

Nutrition: Calories 172, Fats 13.57g, Carbs 6.65g, Net Carbs 3.65g, Protein 5.76g

Zucchini Parmesan Chaffles

Preparation: 5 Minutes | Cooking: 14 Minutes | Servings: 2

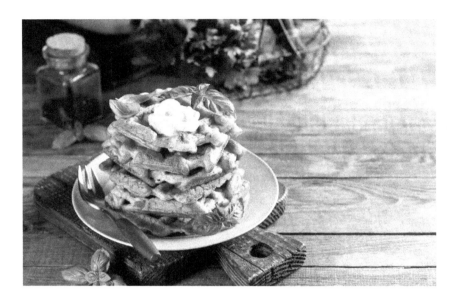

Ingredients

- 1 cup shredded zucchini
- 1 egg, beaten
- ½ cup finely grated Parmesan cheese
- Salt and freshly ground black pepper to taste

Directions

- Preheat the waffle iron.
- Put all the ingredients in a medium bowl and mix well.
- Open the iron and add half of the mixture. Close and cook until crispy, 7 minutes.
- Remove the chaffle onto a plate and make another with the remaining mixture.

- Cut each chaffle into wedges and serve afterward.

Nutrition: Calories 138, Fats 9.07g, Carbs 3.81g, Net Carbs 3.71g, Protein 10.02g

Cheeseburger Chaffle

Cooking: 15 Minutes | Servings: 2

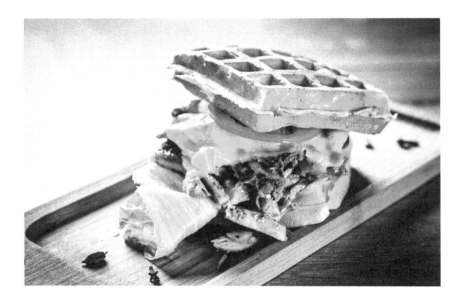

Ingredients

- 1 lb. ground beef
- 1 onion, minced
- 1 tsp. parsley, chopped
- 1 egg, beaten
- Salt and pepper to taste
- 1 tablespoon olive oil
- 4 basic chaffles (Choose 1 Recipe From Chapter 1)
- 2 lettuce leaves
- 2 cheese slices
- 1 tablespoon dill pickles
- Ketchup
- Mayonnaise

54

Directions

- In a large bowl, combine the ground beef, onion, parsley, egg, salt and pepper.
- Mix well.
- Form 2 thick patties.
- Add olive oil to the pan.
- Place the pan over medium heat.
- Cook the patty for 3 to 5 minutes per side or until fully cooked.
- Place the patty on top of each chaffle.
- Top with lettuce, cheese and pickles.
- Squirt ketchup and mayo over the patty and veggies.
- Top with another chaffle.

Nutrition: Calories 325, Total Fat 16.3g, Carbohydrate 3g, Sugars 1.4g, Protein 39.6g

Buffalo Hummus Beef Chaffles

Cooking: 32 Minutes | Servings: 4

Ingredients

- 2 eggs
- 1 cup + ¼ cup finely grated cheddar cheese, divided
- 2 chopped fresh scallions
- Salt and freshly ground black pepper to taste
- 2 chicken breasts, cooked and diced
- ¼ cup buffalo sauce
- 3 tbsp low-carb hummus
- 2 celery stalks, chopped
- ¼ cup crumbled blue cheese for topping

Directions

1. Preheat the waffle iron.
2. In a medium bowl, mix the eggs, 1 cup of the cheddar cheese, scallions, salt, and black pepper,
3. Open the iron and add a quarter of the mixture. Close and cook until crispy, 7 minutes.
4. Transfer the chaffle to a plate and make 3 more chaffles in the same manner.
5. Preheat the oven to 400 F and line a baking sheet with parchment paper. Set aside.
6. Cut the chaffles into quarters and arrange on the baking sheet.
7. In a medium bowl, mix the chicken with the buffalo sauce, hummus, and celery.

8. Spoon the chicken mixture onto each quarter of chaffles and top with the remaining cheddar cheese.
9. Place the baking sheet in the oven and bake until the cheese melts, 4 minutes.
10. Remove from the oven and top with the blue cheese.
11. Serve afterward.

Nutrition: Calories 552, Fats 28.37g, Carbs 6.97g, Net Carbs 6.07g, Protein 59.8g

Brie and Blackberry Chaffles

Cooking: 36 Minutes | Servings: 4

Ingredients
For the chaffles:
- 2 eggs, beaten
- 1 cup finely grated mozzarella cheese

For the topping:
- 1 ½ cups blackberries
- 1 lemon, 1 tsp zest and 2 tbsp juice
- 1 tbsp erythritol
- 4 slices Brie cheese

Directions

For the chaffles:

1. Preheat the waffle iron.
2. Meanwhile, in a medium bowl, mix the eggs and mozzarella cheese.
3. Open the iron, pour in a quarter of the mixture, cover, and cook until crispy, 7 minutes.
4. Remove the chaffle onto a plate and make 3 more with the remaining batter.
5. Plate and set aside.

For the topping:

1. In a medium pot, add the blackberries, lemon zest, lemon juice, and erythritol. Cook until the blackberries break and the sauce thickens, 5 minutes. Turn the heat off.

2. Arrange the chaffles on the baking sheet and place two Brie cheese slices on each. Top with blackberry mixture and transfer the baking sheet to the oven.
3. Bake until the cheese melts, 2 to 3 minutes.
4. Remove from the oven, allow cooling and serve afterward.

Nutrition: Calories 576, Fats 42.22g, Carbs 7.07g, Net Carbs 3.67g, Protein 42.35g

Katsu Chaffles

Preparation: 10 min | Cooking: 5 min | Servings: 2

Ingredients

- Mozzarella cheese (shredded) – 1 cup
- Eggs – 2
- Lettuce (optional) – 2 leaves

For sauce:

- Ketchup (sugar free) – 2 tablespoons
- Oyster sauce – 1 tablespoon
- Worcestershire/Worcester sauce – 2 tablespoons
- Monk fruit/swerve – 1 teaspoon

For chicken:

- Chicken thigh (boneless) – 2 pieces
- Almond flour – 1 cup
- Salt (as desired)
- Eggs – 1
- Black pepper – (as desired)
- Vegetable cooking oil – 2 cups
- Pork rinds – 3 oz.
- Brine
- Salt – 1 tablespoon
- Water – 2 cups

Directions

1. Boil chicken for 30 min then pat it dry
2. Add black pepper and salt to the chicken

3. Mix oyster sauce, Worcestershire sauce, ketchup and Swerve/Monkfruit in one bowl then set aside
4. Grind pork rinds into fine crumbs
5. In separate bowls, add the almond flour, beaten eggs and the crushed pork then coat your chicken pieces using these ingredients in their listed order
6. Fry coated chicken till golden brown
7. Pre-heat and grease waffle maker
8. Mix eggs and Mozzarella cheese together in a bowl
9. Pour into waffle maker and cooking till crunchy
10. Wash and dry green lettuces
11. Spread previously prepared sauces on one chaffle, place some lettuce, one chicken katsu then adds one more chaffle.

Nutrition: Calories 286, Fat 2, Carbs 23, Protein 17

Turkey Chaffle Burger

Cooking: 10 Minutes | Servings: 2

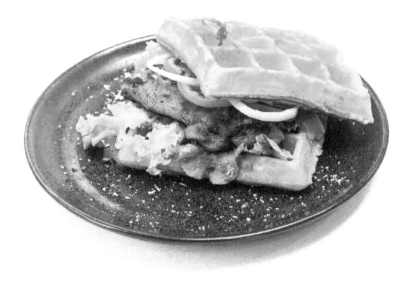

Ingredients

- 2 cups ground turkey
- Salt and pepper to taste
- 1 tablespoon olive oil
- 4 garlic chaffles
- 1 cup Romaine lettuce, chopped
- 1 tomato, sliced
- Mayonnaise
- Ketchup

Directions

1. Combine ground turkey, salt and pepper.
2. Form thick burger patties.
3. Add the olive oil to a pan over medium heat.
4. Cook the turkey burger until fully cooked on both sides.
5. Spread mayo on the chaffle.
6. Top with the turkey burger, lettuce and tomato.
7. Squirt ketchup on top before topping with another chaffle.

Nutrition: Calories 555 Total Fat 21.5g Carbohydrate 4.1g Protein 31.7g Total Sugars 1g

Guacamole Chaffle Bites

Cooking: 14 Minutes | Servings: 2

Ingredients

- 1 large turnip, cooked and mashed
- 2 bacon slices, cooked and finely chopped
- ½ cup finely grated Monterey Jack cheese
- 1 egg, beaten
- 1 cup guacamole for topping

Directions

1. Preheat the waffle iron.
2. Mix all the ingredients except for the guacamole in a medium bowl.
3. Open the iron and add half of the mixture. Close and cook for 4 minutes. Open the lid, flip the chaffle and cook further until golden brown and crispy, minutes.
4. Remove the chaffle onto a plate and make another in the same manner.
5. Cut each chaffle into wedges, top with the guacamole and serve afterward.

Nutrition: Calories 311 Fats 22.52g Carbs 8.29g Net Carbs 5.79g Protein 13.g

Chaffle Chicken Breast Stuffed with Spinach, Pine Nuts, and Feta

Preparation:20 minutes | Cooking: 15 minutes | Servings: 4-6

Ingredients

- 1 cup finely chopped fresh baby spinach
- 3/4 cup feta cheese, crumbled
- 2 tablespoons toasted pine nuts
- 2 cloves garlic, minced
- ½ teaspoon dried thyme
- 4 boneless, skinless chicken breast halves
- ½ teaspoon salt
- ½ teaspoon freshly ground black pepper
- **NOTE:** The Use of baby spinach reduces the stress of picking through to remove large stems.
- The use of toasted pine nut is to bring out the flavor.

Directions

1. Toasting the pine nut
2. Put the pine nuts inside a dry pan over medium heat.
3. Stir frequently till the nuts become fragrant and are barely turning brown.
4. Remove from the heat and pour them onto a plate to cool.

Making the Chaffles

1. Preheat the waffle iron and oven on medium.
2. Put the spinach, cheese, nuts, garlic, and thyme in a small bowl.

3. Smash together until the filling becomes cohesive and easier to handle.
4. Lightly grease the waffle iron
5. Make a parallel cut into the thickest portion of each chicken breast half to form a pocket. But do not to cut through.
6. Divide the combination into four equal parts and fill up each pocket in the chicken breasts, leaving a margin at the edge to close.
7. Season the chicken with salt and pepper.
8. Arrange the chicken into the waffle iron to allow lid to press down on the chicken more evenly.
9. Close the lid.
10. Cooking the chicken for 8 minutes. Check and rotate if need be and cooking for about 3 minutes. The chicken should be golden brown.
11. Remove the chicken from the waffle iron
12. Repeat baking procedure with any remaining chicken.
13. Keep cooked chicken warm and serve warm.

Nutrition: Calories 158, Fat 13.3, Fiber 3.9, Carbs 8.9, Protein 3.3

Chicken and Chaffle Nachos

Cooking: 33 Minutes | Servings: 4

Ingredients

For the chaffles:

- 2 eggs, beaten
- 1 cup finely grated Mexican cheese blend

For the topping:

- 2 tbsp butter
- 1 tbsp almond flour
- ¼ cup unsweetened almond milk
- 1 cup finely grated cheddar cheese + more to garnish
- 3 bacon slices, cooked and chopped
- 2 cups cooked and diced chicken breasts
- 2 tbsp hot sauce
- 2 tbsp chopped fresh scallions

Directions

For the chaffles:

1. Preheat the waffle iron.
2. In a medium bowl, mix the eggs and Mexican cheese blend.
3. Open the iron and add a quarter of the mixture. Close and cook until crispy, 7 minutes.
4. Transfer the chaffle to a plate and make 3 more chaffles in the same manner.

5. Place the chaffles on serving plates and set aside for serving.

For the chicken-cheese topping:

6. Melt the butter in a large skillet and mix in the almond flour until brown, 1 minute.
7. Pour the almond milk and whisk until well combined. Simmer until thickened, 2 minutes.
8. Stir in the cheese to melt, 2 minutes and then mix in the bacon, chicken, and hot sauce.
9. Spoon the mixture onto the chaffles and top with some more cheddar cheese.
10. Garnish with the scallions and serve immediately.

Nutrition: Calories 524 Fats 37.51g Carbs 3.55g Net Carbs 3.25g Protein 41.86g

Ham, Cheese & Tomato Chaffle Sandwich

Cooking: 10 Minutes | Servings: 2

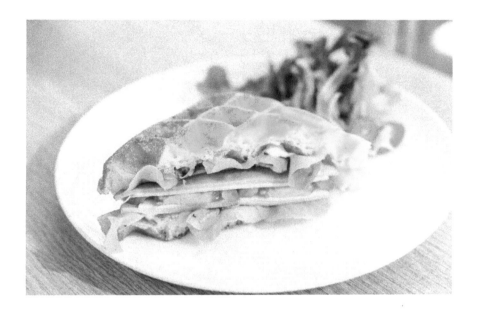

Ingredients

- 1 teaspoon olive oil
- 2 slices ham
- 4 basic chaffles (Choose 1 Recipe from Chapter 1)
- 1 tablespoon mayonnaise
- 2 slices Provolone cheese
- 1 tomato, sliced

Directions

- Add the olive oil to a pan over medium heat.
- Cook the ham for 1 minute per side.

- Spread the chaffles with mayonnaise.
- Top with the ham, cheese and tomatoes.
- Top with another chaffle to make a sandwich.
- Nutrition value:
- Calories 198 Fat 14.7g Carbohydrate 4.6g Sugars 1.5g Protein 12.2g

Eggs Benedict Chaffle

Preparation: 20 min. | Cooking: 10 min. | Servings: 2

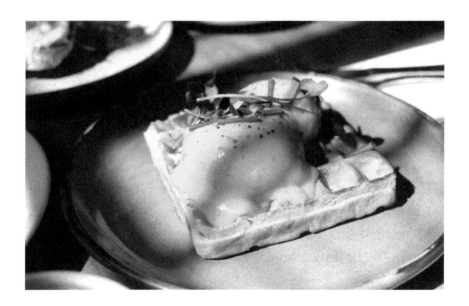

Ingredients

For the chaffle:

- 2 egg whites
- 2 Tbsp almond flour
- 1 Tbsp sour cream
- ½ cup mozzarella cheese

For the hollandaise:

- ½ cup salted butter
- 4 egg yolks
- 2 Tbsp lemon juice

For the poached eggs:

- 2 eggs
- 1 Tbsp white vinegar
- 3 oz deli ham

Directions:

1. Whip egg white until frothy, then mix in remaining ingredients. Turn on waffle maker to heat and oil it with cooking spray.
2. Cook for 7 minutes until golden brown.
3. Remove chaffle and repeat with remaining batter. Fill half the pot with water and bring to a boil.
4. Place heat-safe bowl on top of pot, ensuring bottom doesn't touch the boiling water. Heat butter to boiling in a microwave.
5. Add yolks to double boiler bowl and bring to boil.
6. Add hot butter to the bowl and whisk briskly. Cook until the egg yolk mixture has thickened.
7. Remove bowl from pot and add in lemon juice. Set aside.
8. Add more water to pot if needed to make the poached eggs (water should completely cover the eggs).
9. Bring to a simmer. Add white vinegar to water.
10. Crack eggs into simmering water and cook for 1 minute 30 seconds. Remove using slotted spoon.
11. Warm chaffles in toaster for 2-3 minutes. Top with ham, poached eggs, and hollandaise sauce.

Nutrition: Carbs: 4 g, Fat: 26 g, Protein: 26 g, Calories: 365

Cheddar Jalapeño Chaffle

Preparation: 5 min. | Cooking: 5 min. | Servings: 2

Ingredients

- 2 large eggs
- ½ cup shredded mozzarella
- ¼ cup almond flour
- ½ tsp baking powder
- ¼ cup shredded cheddar cheese
- 2 Tbsp diced jalapeños jarred or canned

For the toppings:

- ½ cooked bacon, chopped
- 2 Tbsp cream cheese
- ¼ jalapeño slices

Directions

1. Turn on waffle maker to heat and oil it with cooking spray.
2. Mix mozzarella, eggs, baking powder, almond flour, and garlic powder in a bowl. Sprinkle 2 Tbsp cheddar cheese in a thin layer on waffle maker, and ½ jalapeño. Ladle half of the egg mixture on top of the cheese and jalapeños.
3. Cook for 5 minutes, or until done. Repeat for the second chaffle.
4. Top with cream cheese, bacon, and jalapeño slices.

Nutrition: Carbs: 5 g, Fat: 18 g, Protein: 18 g, Calories: 307

Broccoli and Cheese Chaffles

Preparation: 5 min. | Cooking: 5 min. | Servings: 1

Ingredients

- ⅓ cup raw broccoli, finely chopped
- ¼ cup shredded cheddar cheese
- 1 egg
- ½ tsp garlic powder
- ½ tsp dried minced onion
- Salt and pepper, to taste

Directions

1. Turn on waffle maker to heat and oil it with cooking spray. Beat egg in a small bowl.
2. Fold in cheese, broccoli, onion, garlic powder, salt, and pepper. Pour egg mixture into waffle maker. Cook for 4 minutes, or until done. Remove from waffle maker with a fork.
3. Serve with sour cream or butter.

Nutrition: Carbs: 4 g, Fat: 9 g, Protein: 7 g, Calories: 125

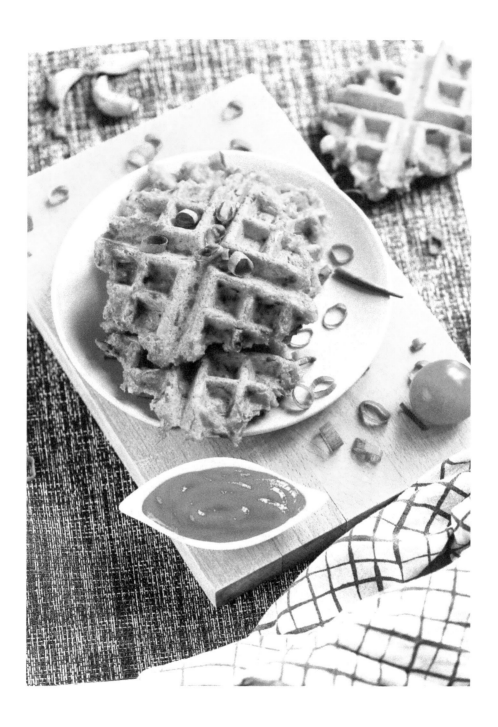

Chapter 4: Vegan and Vegetarian Recipes

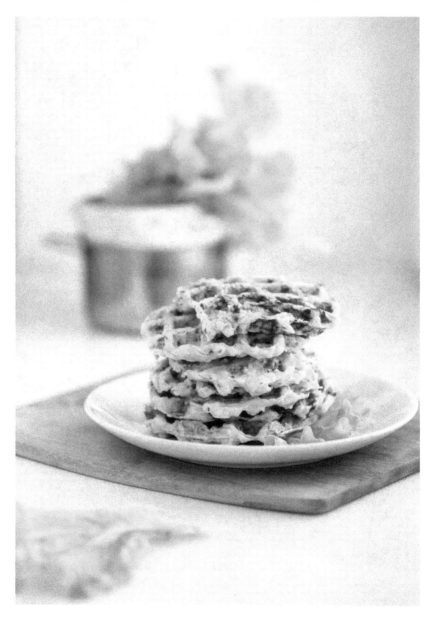

Vegan Chocolate Chaffles

Servings: 2 | Cooking: 5minutes

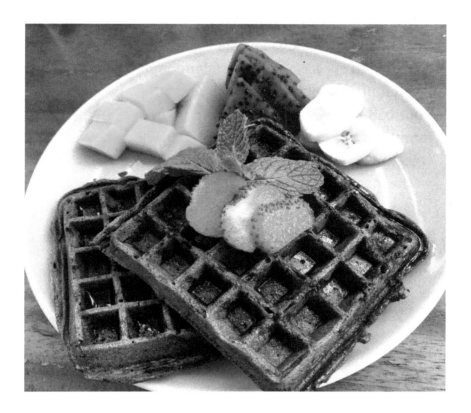

Ingredients

- 1/2 cupcoconut flour
- 3 tbsps. cocoa powder
- 2 tbsps. whole psyllium husk
- 1/2 teaspoon baking powder
- pinch of salt
- 1/2 cup vegan cheese, softened
- 1/4 cup coconut milk

Directions

1. Prepare your waffle iron according to the manufacturer's Directions.
2. Mix together coconut flour, cocoa powder, baking powder, salt and husk in a bowl and set aside.
3. Add melted cheese and milk and mix well. Let it stand for a few minutes before cooking.
4. Pour batter in waffle machine and cook for about 3-minutesutes.
5. Once chaffles are cooked, carefully remove them from the waffle machine.
6. Serve with vegan icecream and enjoy!

Nutrition: Protein: 32% 42 kcal, Fat: 63% 82 kcal, Carbohydrates: 5% 6 kcal

Apple Cinnamon Chaffles

Preparation: 6 minutes | Cooking: 20 Minutes | Servings: 2

Ingredients
- 3 eggs, lightly beaten
- 1 cup mozzarella cheese, shredded
- ¼ cup apple, chopped
- ½ tsp monk fruit sweetener
- 1 ½ tsp cinnamon
- ¼ tsp baking powder, gluten-free
- 2 tbsp coconut flour

Directions
1. Preheat your waffle maker.
2. Add all ingredients in a medium bowl and stir until well combined.
3. Spray waffle maker with cooking spray.
4. Pour 1/3 of batter in the hot waffle maker and cook for minutes or until golden brown. Repeat with the remaining batter.
5. Serve and enjoy.

Nutrition: Calories 227, Fat 18.6, Fiber 4.5, Carbs 9.5, Protein 9.9

Blueberry Chaffles

Preparation: 8 minutes | Cooking: 15 Minutes | Servings: 2

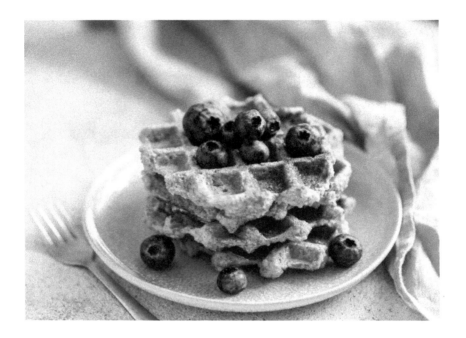

Ingredients

- 2 eggs
- 1/2 cup blueberries
- 1/2 tsp baking powder
- 1/2 tsp vanilla
- 2 tsp Swerve
- 3 tbsp almond flour
- 1 cup mozzarella cheese, shredded

Directions

1. Preheat your waffle maker.

2. In a medium bowl, mix eggs, vanilla, Swerve, almond flour, and cheese.
3. Add blueberries and stir well.
4. Spray waffle maker with cooking spray.
5. Pour 1/4 batter in the hot waffle maker and cook for 8 minutes or until golden brown. Repeat with the remaining batter.
6. Serve and enjoy.

Nutrition: Calories 96, Fat 6.1g, Carbohydrates 5g, Sugar 2.2g, Protein 6.1g, Cholesterol 86 mg

Vegetarian Chaffle Sandwich

Cooking: 8 Minutes | Servings: 2

Ingredients

Chaffle:

- 1 large egg (beaten)
- 1/8 tsp onion powder
- 1 tbsp almond flour
- 1/2 cup shredded mozzarella cheese
- 1 tsp nutmeg
- 1/4 tsp baking powder

Sandwich Filling:

- 1/2 cup shredded carrot
- 1/2 cup sliced cucumber
- 1/2 medium bell pepper (sliced)
- 1 cup mixed salad greens
- 1/2 avocado (mashed and divided)
- 6 tbsp keto friendly hummus

Directions

For the chaffle:

1. Plug the waffle maker to preheat it. Spray it with non-stick cooking spray.
2. Combine the baking powder, nutmeg, flour and onion powder in a mixing bowl. Add the eggs and mix.

3. Add the cheese and mix until the ingredients are well combined and you have formed a smooth batter.
4. Pour the batter into the waffle maker and spread it out to the edges of the waffle maker to cover all the holes on it.
5. Close the waffle lid and cook for about 5 minutes or according to waffle maker's settings.
6. After the cooking cycle, remove the chaffle from the waffle maker with a plastic or silicone utensil.

For the sandwich:

7. Add 3 tablespoons of hummus to one chaffle and spread with a spoon.
8. Fill another chaffle with one half of the mashed avocado.
9. Fill the first chaffle slice with 1/4 cup sliced cucumber, 1/2 cup mixed salad greens, 1/4 cup shredded carrot and
10. one half of the sliced bell pepper.
11. Place the chaffle on top and press lightly.
12. Repeat step 7 to 10 for the remaining ingredients to make the second sandwich.
13. Serve and enjoy.

Nutrition: Fat 22g 28%, Carbohydrate 17.8g 6%, Sugars 4.6g, Protein 11.3g

Garlic Mayo Vegan Chaffles

Cooking: 5minutes | Servings: 2

Ingredients

- 1 tbsp. chia seeds
- 2 ½ tbsps. water
- ¼ cup low carb vegan cheese
- 2 tbsps. coconut flour
- 1 cup low carb vegan cream cheese, softened
- 1 tsp. garlic powder
- pinch of salt
- 2 tbsps. vegan garlic mayo for topping

Directions

1. Preheat your square waffle maker.
2. In a small bowl, mix chia seeds and water, let it stand for 5 minutes.
3. Add all ingredients to the chia seeds mixture and mix well.
4. Pour vegan chaffle batter in a greased waffle maker
5. Close the waffle maker and cook for about 3-minutesutes.
6. Once chaffles are cooked, remove from the maker.
7. Top with garlic mayo and pepper.
8. Enjoy!

Nutrition: Protein: 32% 42 kcal, Fat: 63% 82 kcal, Carbohydrates: 5% 6 kcal

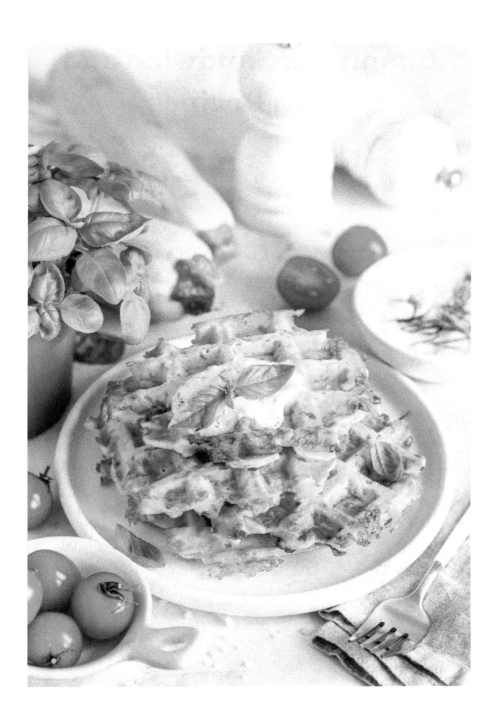

Chapter 5: Sandwich and Pizza Recipes

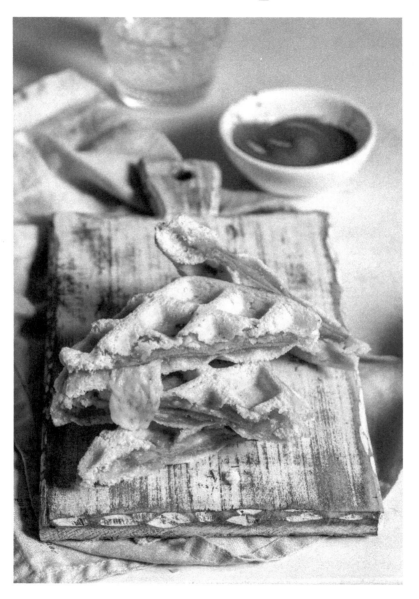

Ham and Parmesan Pizza Chaffle

Preparation: 5 minutes | Cooking: 13 minutes | Servings: 2 pizza chaffles

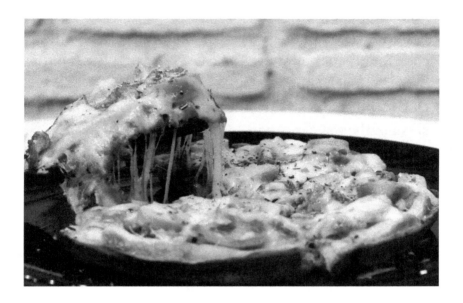

Ingredients

For chaffles

- ½ cup shredded mozzarella cheese
- 1 tbsp almond flour
- ½ tsp baking powder
- 1 egg, beaten

For topping:

- 2 tbsp low carb pasta sauce
- 2 tbsp mozzarella cheese
- 1 tbsp parmesan cheese
- 2 slices of ham

Directions

1. Heat up the waffle maker.
2. Add mozzarella cheese, baking powder, egg, and almond flour to a medium mixing bowl and combine well.
3. Pour down half of the batter into the waffle maker and cook for about 4 minutes. Repeat now with the rest of the batter to make another chaffle.
4. Once both chaffles are cooked, place them on the baking sheet of the toaster oven.
5. Put 1 tbsp of low carb pasta sauce on top of each pizza chaffle.
6. Sprinkle 1 tbsp of shredded mozzarella cheese on top of each one.
7. Top with a slice of ham and sprinkle with parmesan cheese.
8. Bake it at 350° in the toaster oven for about 5 minutes, until the cheese is melted.
9. Serve and enjoy!

Broccoli Pizza Chaffle

Preparation: 5 minutes | Cooking: 10 minutes | Servings: 2 chaffles

Ingredients

For chaffles:

- ½ cup shredded mozzarella cheese
- 1 tbsp almond flour
- ½ tsp baking powder
- 1 egg, beaten
- ½ tsp garlic powder
- A pinch of salt

For topping:

- 2 tbsp low carb pasta sauce
- 2 tbsp mozzarella cheese, shredded
- 2 tbsp broccoli, boiled and chopped

Directions

1. Heat up the waffle maker.
2. Add all the chaffle ingredients to a small mixing bowl and combine well.
3. Pour down half of the batter into the waffle maker and cook for about 4 minutes until golden brown. Repeat now with the rest of the batter to make another chaffle.
4. Once both chaffles are cooked, place them on the baking sheet of the toaster oven.
5. Put 1 tbsp of low carb pasta sauce on top of each chaffle.

6. Sprinkle 1 tbsp of shredded mozzarella cheese on top of each one.
7. Top with broccoli.
8. Bake it at 350° in the toaster oven for about 2 minutes, until the cheese is melted.
9. Serve and enjoy!

Veggie Pizza Chaffle

Preparation: 5 minutes | Cooking: 13 minutes | Servings: 2 chaffles

Ingredients

For chaffles:

- ½ cup shredded mozzarella cheese
- 1 tbsp almond flour
- ½ tsp baking powder
- 1 egg, beaten
- ¼ tsp garlic powder
- A pinch of salt and pepper

For pizza topping:

- 2 tbsp low carb pasta sauce
- 2 tbsp mozzarella cheese, shredded
- ½ tbsp onion, browned and chopped
- ½ tbsp mushrooms, chopped
- ½ tbsp zucchini, grated
- ¼ tsp fresh basil

Directions

1. Heat up the waffle maker.
2. Add all the chaffle ingredients to a small mixing bowl and combine well.
3. Pour down half of the batter into the waffle maker and cook for about 4 minutes until golden brown. Repeat now with the rest of the batter to make another chaffle.

4. Once both chaffles are cooked, place them on the baking sheet of the toaster oven.
5. Put 1 tbsp of low carb pasta sauce on top of each chaffle.
6. Sprinkle 1 tbsp of shredded mozzarella on top of each one. Season with fresh basil.
7. Top the chaffle with onions, zucchinis and mushrooms.
8. Bake it at 350° in the toaster oven for about 5 minutes, until the cheese is melted.
9. Serve and enjoy!

Ham and Zucchini Pizza Chaffle

Preparation: 5 minutes | Cooking: 10 minutes | Servings: 2 chaffles

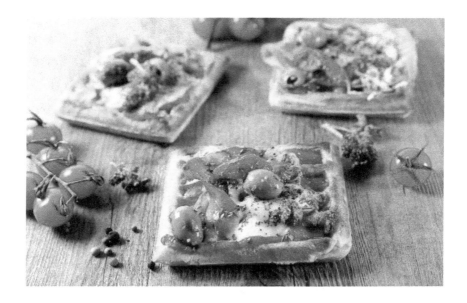

Ingredients

For chaffles:

- ½ cup shredded mozzarella cheese
- 1 tbsp almond flour
- ½ tsp baking powder
- 1 egg, beaten
- A pinch of salt

For topping:

- 2 tbsp low carb pasta sauce
- 2 tbsp mozzarella cheese, shredded

- 2 slices of ham
- 2 tbsp zucchini, grated

Directions

1. Heat up the waffle maker.
2. Add all the chaffle ingredients to a small mixing bowl and combine well.
3. Pour down half of the batter into the waffle maker and cook for about 4 minutes until golden brown color. Repeat now with the rest of the batter to make another chaffle.
4. Once both chaffles are cooked, place them on the baking sheet of the toaster oven.
5. Put 1 tbsp of low carb pasta sauce on top of each chaffle.
6. Sprinkle 1 tbsp of shredded mozzarella cheese on top of each one.
7. Top with a slice of ham and zucchinis.
8. Bake it at 350° in the toaster oven for about 2 minutes, until the cheese is melted.
9. Serve and enjoy!

Spicy Pizza Chaffle

Preparation: 5 minutes | Cooking: 10 minutes | Servings: 2 chaffles

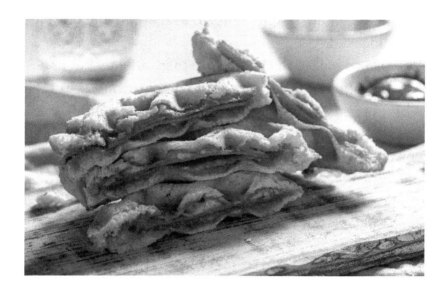

Ingredients

For chaffles:

- ½ cup shredded mozzarella cheese
- 1 tbsp almond flour
- ½ tsp baking powder
- 1 egg, beaten
- ½ tsp hot pepper powder
- A pinch of salt

For topping:

- 2 tbsp low carb pasta sauce
- 2 tbsp mozzarella cheese, shredded

95

- 1 tsp fresh parsley

Directions

1. Heat up the waffle maker.
2. Add all the chaffle ingredients to a small mixing bowl and combine well.
3. Pour down half of the batter into the waffle maker and cook for about 4 minutes until golden brown. Repeat now with the rest of the batter to make another chaffle.
4. Once both chaffles are cooked, place them on the baking sheet of the toaster oven.
5. Put 1 tbsp of low carb pasta sauce on top of each chaffle.
6. Sprinkle 1 tbsp of shredded mozzarella cheese on top of each one. Season with parsley.
7. Bake it at 350° in the toaster oven for about 2 minutes, until the cheese is melted.
8. Serve and enjoy!

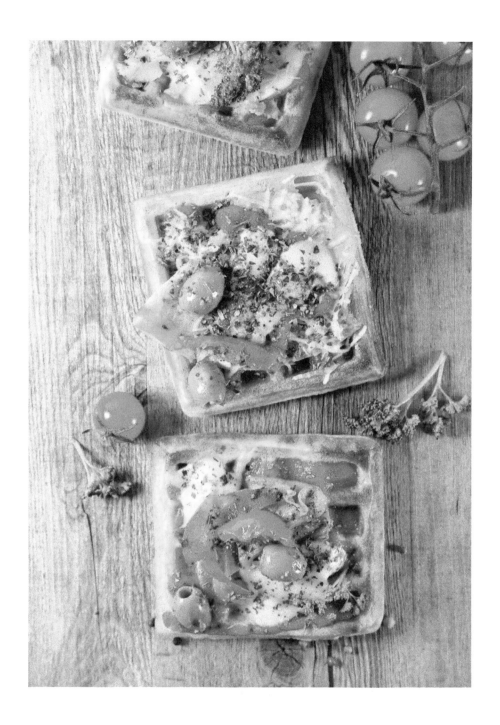

Chapter 6: Sweet and Dessert Recipes

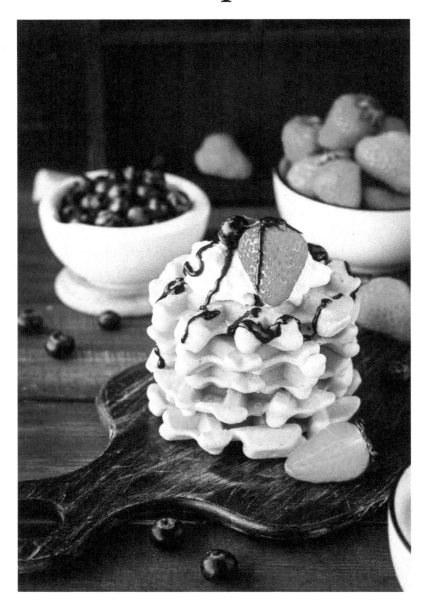

Chocolate Chips Chaffle

Preparation: 4 minutes | Cooking: 8 minutes | Servings: 2 chaffles

Ingredients

- ½ cup shredded mozzarella cheese
- 1 tbsp almond flour
- 1 egg
- ¼ tsp cinnamon
- ½ tbsp sweetener
- 2 tbsp low carb chocolate chips

Directions

1. Heat up the waffle maker.
2. Now, mix the mozzarella cheese, almond flour, egg, cinnamon, sweetener and chocolate chips in a small mixing bowl.
3. Add half of the batter into the waffle maker and cook it for approx. 4-5 min. When the first one is completely done cooking, cook the second one.
4. Set aside for 1-2 minutes.
5. Serve and enjoy!

Chocolate Chips Chaffle Nr. 2

Preparation: 5 minutes | Cooking: 8 minutes | Servings: 2 chaffles

Ingredients

- 1 egg
- ½ cup shredded mozzarella cheese
- 1 tbsp whipping cream
- ½ tsp coconut flour
- ¼ tsp baking powder
- A pinch of salt
- 1 tbsp chocolate chips, unsweetened

Directions

1. Heat up the waffle maker.
2. Mix all the ingredients except the chocolate chips in a small mixing bowl.
3. Grease waffle maker, then pour half of the batter onto the bottom plate of the waffle maker. Sprinkle now a few chocolate chips on top and then close.
4. Cook for approx. 4 minutes or until the chaffle is golden brown.
5. Repeat now with the rest of the batter.
6. Let chaffle sit for a few minutes so that it begins to crisp.
7. Serve with sugar-free whipped topping and enjoy!

Chocolate Chips Chaffle Nr. 3

Preparation: 5 minutes | Cooking: 8 minutes | Servings: 2 chaffles

Ingredients

- 2 tsp coconut flour
- 2 tbsp sweetener
- 1 tbsp cocoa powder
- ¼ tsp baking powder
- 1 egg
- ½ cup shredded mozzarella cheese
- 1 tbsp cream cheese
- ½ tsp vanilla extract
- 1 tbsp unsweetened chocolate chips

Directions

1. Heat up the waffle maker.
2. In a small mixing bowl, beat egg.
3. Add all the other ingredients, except for chocolate chips, and combine well.
4. Pour half of the batter onto the bottom plate of the waffle maker. Sprinkle now a few chocolate chips on top and then close.
5. Cook now for approx. 4 min or until the chaffle is golden brown.
6. Repeat with the rest of the batter.
7. Serve with your favorite berries and enjoy!

Keto Chocolate Chaffle

Preparation: 5 minutes | Cooking: 8 minutes | Servings: 2 chaffles

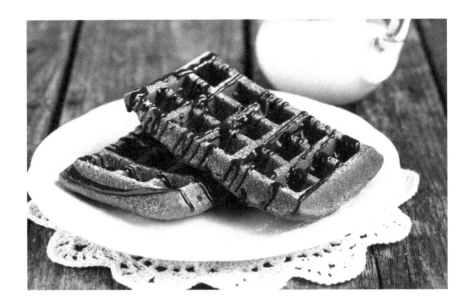

Ingredients

- 1 large egg
- ½ cup Gruyere cheese, shredded
- 1 tsp almond flour
- ¼ tsp vanilla extract
- 1 tsp heavy whipping cream
- 2 tbsp cocoa powder, unsweetened
- ¼ tsp baking powder
- 2 tbsp sweetener
- Salt to taste

Directions

1. Heat up the waffle maker.
2. Now, add all the ingredients to a small mixing bowl and stir until well combined.
3. Now, pour half of the batter onto the bottom plate of the waffle maker.
4. Cook for approx. 4 minutes or until the chaffle is golden brown.
5. Repeat with the rest of the batter.
6. Serve with your favorite berries and enjoy!

Walnut Pumpkin Chaffles

Cooking: 10 Minutes | Servings: 2

Ingredients

- 1 organic egg, beaten
- ½ cup Mozzarella cheese, shredded
- 2 tablespoons almond flour
- 1 tablespoon sugar-free pumpkin puree
- 1 teaspoon Erythritol
- ¼ teaspoon ground cinnamon
- 2 tablespoons walnuts, toasted and chopped

Directions

1. Preheat a mini waffle iron and then grease it.
2. In a bowl, place all ingredients except walnuts and beat until well combined.
3. Fold in the walnuts.
4. Place now half of the mixture into preheated waffle iron and cook for about 5 minutes or until golden brown.
5. Repeat with the remaining mixture.
6. Serve warm.

Nutrition: Calories: 148, Net Carb: 1.6g, Fat: 11.8g, Saturated Fat: 2g, Carbohydrates: 3.3g, Dietary Fiber: 1g, Sugar: 0.8g, Protein: 6.7g

Protein Mozzarella Chaffles

Cooking: 20 Minutes | Servings: 4

Ingredients

- ½ scoop unsweetened protein powder
- 2 large organic eggs
- ½ cup Mozzarella cheese, shredded
- 1 tablespoon Erythritol
- ¼ teaspoon organic vanilla extract

Directions

1. Preheat a mini waffle iron and then grease it.
2. In a medium bowl, place all ingredients and with a fork, mix until well combined.
3. Place ¼ of the mixture into preheated waffle iron and cook for about 4-5 minutes or until golden brown.
4. Repeat with the remaining mixture.
5. Serve warm.

Nutrition: Net Carb: 0.4g, Fat: 3.3g, Saturated Fat: 1.2g, Carbohydrates: 0.4g, Dietary Fiber: 0g, Sugar: 0.2g, Protein: 7.3g

Chocolate Chips Peanut Butter Chaffles

Cooking: 8 Minutes | Servings: 2

Ingredients

- 1 organic egg, beaten
- ¼ cup Mozzarella cheese, shredded
- 2 tablespoons creamy peanut butter
- 1 tablespoon almond flour
- 1 tablespoon granulated Erythritol
- 1 teaspoon organic vanilla extract
- 1 tablespoon 70% dark chocolate chips

Directions

1. Preheat a mini waffle iron and then grease it.
2. In a bowl, place all ingredients except chocolate chips and beat until well combined.
3. Gently, fold in the chocolate chips.
4. Place half of the mixture into preheated waffle iron and cook it for about minutes or until golden brown.
5. Repeat with the remaining mixture.
6. Serve warm.

Nutrition: Calories: 214, Net Carb: 4.1g, Fat: 16.8g, Saturated Fat: 5.4g, Carbohydrates: 6.4g, Dietary Fiber: 2.3g, Sugar: 2.1g, Protein: 8.8g

Pumpkin Chaffles

Cooking: 12 Minutes | Servings: 2

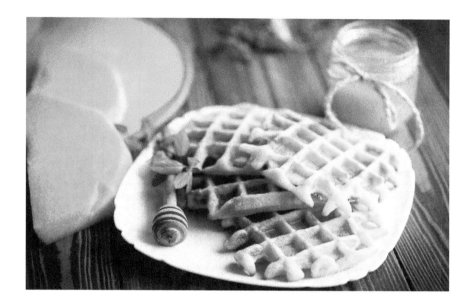

Ingredients

- 1 organic egg, beaten
- ½ cup Mozzarella cheese, shredded
- 1½ tablespoon homemade pumpkin puree
- ½ teaspoon Erythritol
- ½ teaspoon organic vanilla extract
- ¼ teaspoon pumpkin pie spice

Directions

1. Preheat a mini waffle iron and then grease it.
2. In a bowl, place all your ingredients and beat until well combined.

3. Place ¼ of the mixture into preheated waffle iron and cook for about 4-6 minutes or until golden brown.
4. Repeat with the remaining mixture.
5. Serve warm.

Nutrition: Calories: 59, Net Carb: 1.2g, Fat: 3.5g, Saturated Fat: 1.5g, Carbohydrates: 1g, Dietary Fiber: 0.4g, Sugar: 0.7g, Protein: 4.9g

Peanut Butter Chaffles

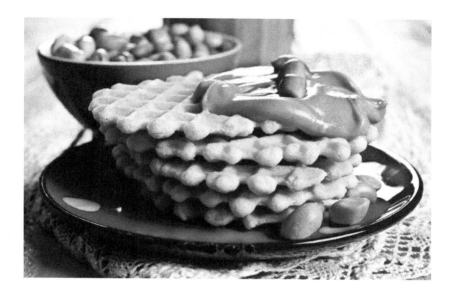

Ingredients

- 1 organic egg, beaten
- ½ cup Mozzarella cheese, shredded
- 3 tablespoons granulated Erythritol
- 2 tablespoons peanut butter

Directions

1. Preheat a mini waffle iron and then grease it.
2. In a medium bowl, place all ingredients and with a fork, mix until well combined.
3. Place half of your mixture into preheated waffle iron and cook for about 4 minutes or until golden brown.
4. Repeat now with the remaining mixture.

5. Serve warm.

Nutrition: Calories: 145, Net Carb: 2g, Fat: 11.5g, Saturated Fat: 3.1g, Carbohydrates: 3.6g, Dietary Fiber: 1g, Sugar: 1.7g, Protein: 8.8g

Almond Butter Chaffles

Cooking: 10 Minutes | Servings: 2

Ingredients

- 1 large organic egg, beaten
- 1/3 cup Mozzarella cheese, shredded
- 1 tablespoon Erythritol
- 2 tablespoons almond butter
- 1 teaspoon organic vanilla extract

Directions

1. Preheat a mini waffle iron and then grease it.
2. In a medium bowl, place all ingredients and with a fork, mix until they are well combined.
3. Place half of the mixture into preheated waffle iron and cook for about 5 minutes or until golden brown.
4. Repeat with the remaining mixture.
5. Serve warm.

Nutrition: Calories: 153, Net Carb: 2g, Fat: 12.3g, Saturated Fat: 2g, Carbohydrates: 3g, Dietary Fiber: 1.6g, Sugar: 1.2g, Protein: 7.9g

Red Chaffle

Preparation: 5 minutes | Cooking: 8 minutes | Servings: 2 chaffles

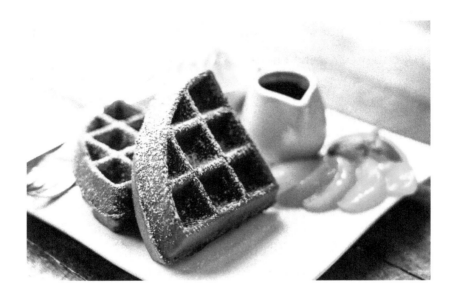

Ingredients

Chaffle:

- 2 tsp processed cocoa
- 2 tsp sweetener
- 1 egg
- ½ cup mozzarella cheese, shredded
- 2 drops red food coloring
- ¼ tsp baking powder
- 1 tbsp heavy whipping cream

For the Frosting:

- 2 tsp sweetener

- 2 tbsp softened cream cheese
- ¼ tsp vanilla

Directions

1. Heat up the waffle maker.
2. Mix the egg and the other ingredients in a small mixing bowl. Mix well until the batter is creamy.
3. Pour now half of the batter into the waffle maker and cook for 4 minutes. Now, repeat with the rest of the batter to make another chaffle.
4. In a separate bowl, add the sweetener, cream cheese, and vanilla. Mix the frosting until well incorporated.
5. Spread the frosting on the chaffles after it has completely cooled.
6. Serve and enjoy!

Cinnamon Chaffle

Preparation: 5 minutes | Cooking: 8 minutes | Servings:　2 chaffles

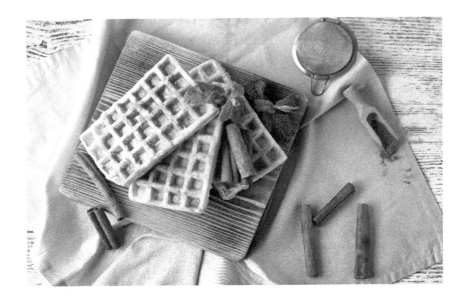

Ingredients

Chaffle:

- 1 egg
- ½ cup mozzarella cheese, shredded
- 2 tbsp almond flour
- 1 tbsp sweetener
- ½ tsp vanilla extract
- ¼ tsp cinnamon
- ½ tsp baking powder

For the Coating:

- 1 tbsp butter
- 2 tbsp sweetener
- ½ tsp cinnamon

Directions

1. Heat up the waffle maker.
2. Add all the chaffles ingredients to a small mixing bowl and mix well until creamy.
3. Pour now half of the batter into the waffle maker and cook for 4 minutes. Now, repeat with the rest of the batter to make another chaffle.
4. Let cool for 3 minutes to let chaffles get crispy.
5. In a bowl, combine sweetener and cinnamon for coating.
6. Melt butter in a microwave safe bowl, brush the chaffles with the butter.
7. Sprinkle sweetener and cinnamon mixture on both sides of the chaffles once they're brushed with butter.
8. Serve and enjoy!

Chocolate Peanut Butter Chaffle

Preparation: 4 minutes | Cooking: 8 minutes | Servings: 2 chaffles

Ingredients

- 1 egg, beaten
- ½ cup mozzarella cheese, shredded
- 2 tbsp almond flour
- ¼ tsp sweetener
- 1 tbsp unsweetened powdered cocoa
- ¼ tsp baking powder
- 2 tbsp unsweetened keto approved peanut butter

Directions

1. Heat up the waffle maker.
2. Now, add all the ingredients to a small mixing bowl. Stir well.
3. Now, pour half of the batter into the waffle maker and cook for 4 minutes until you see golden brown color. Repeat with the rest of the batter to make another chaffle.
4. Serve and enjoy!

Cinnamon and Pumpkin Chaffle

Preparation: 5 minutes | Cooking: 8 minutes | Servings: 2 chaffles

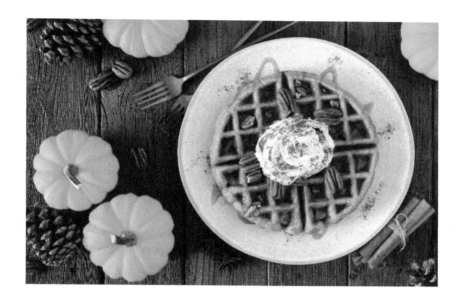

Ingredients

Chaffle:

- 1 egg
- ½ cup mozzarella cheese, shredded
- 3 tbsp coconut flour
- 1 tsp baking powder
- ¼ cup pumpkin puree
- ½ tsp pumpkin spice seasoning
- 1 tsp vanilla extract
- A pinch of salt
- 1 tbsp cinnamon powder

Topping:

- 2 tbsp maple syrup, unsweetened

Directions

1. Heat up the waffle maker.
2. Add all the chaffles ingredients to a small mixing bowl and stir until well combined.
3. Pour now half of the batter into the waffle maker and cook for 4 minutes until you see golden brown color. Repeat with the rest of the batter to make another chaffle.
4. Let cool for 3 minutes to let chaffles get crispy.
5. Top with maple syrup.
6. Serve and enjoy!

CPSIA information can be obtained
at www.ICGtesting.com
Printed in the USA
BVHW092310270421
605945BV00010B/1146

9 781911 688204